MASSAGE

FOR HEALTH

By

MIRKA KNASTER

HEALING ARTS
HOME VIDEO

Not all of the massage instruction presented in this book and accompanying video are suitable to everyone. To reduce the risk of injury consult your doctor before beginning the massage program. The following instructions are in no way intended as a substitute for medical counseling. The author and the publisher disclaim any liability or loss, personal or otherwise, resulting from the procedures in this book and video.

Book Design by Christine Wilson

Cover Photograph Mario Casilli

Manufactured in the United States of America

FOREWORD

Several years ago I had my first opportunity to work overseas on a commercial modeling assignment in exotic Japan. Not knowing what to expect, I ran straight out and bought "Shogun" to prepare myself for this exciting adventure. And what an adventure it was—a wonderful experience! But, what James Clavell's book hadn't prepared me for was how stressful it would be.

For two weeks, I was working twelve hour days under sweltering lights with every kind of noise and foreign language imaginable thundering all around me. All the while my mind was reeling: Why had I come?...Was my husband OK?...Was I what they wanted?...Was this what I wanted?... In no time at all I had managed to tighten every muscle in my body as taut as a well-made military bunk.

A young Japanese woman I befriended suggested I get a massage. Well, normally I would have brushed aside the suggestion, but instead I thought what a perfect idea! Experiencing a Japanese style "Shiatsu" massage turned out to be one of the best gifts I have ever given myself....

From the moment I walked into the room, I knew this was going to be a positive experience...soothing Japanese pipe music was playing, the air was warm and cozy, and the masseuse was unhurried and relaxed. I found my mind starting to clear. With every stroke I could feel all the tension in my back, shoulders and neck escaping through her fingertips. During the remainder of my trip, I went back three times, and have be come a sworn believer in the benefits of massage ever since.

Over the years I have come to find that a great number of my friends and co-workers also consider massage to be a saving grace in their hectic routines. Whether it's feet, temples, backs or full body, "getting a rub down" has become as much a positive part of their lives as exercise. And yet, some people still have questions about it. So that's why I've tried to take some of the mystery out of massage by creating a step-by-step instruction that shows just how easy it is to learn— and how marvelous it is to receive. With the help of massage experts Mirka Knaster, and James Heartland "Massage For Health" will give you the opportunity to discover the rewards of massage in the privacy of your own home.

I think you'll agree with the millions of people who already utilize massage, it's fun, and a healthy way to reduce the effects of stress. Once I learned how to give a massage, I couldn't wait to offer an aching shoulder a bit of relief. Give the gift of massage to yourself or someone you love. You're worth it!

PREFACE

When I bought my first massage book about fifteen years ago and tried to practice on a friend, I never knew if I was really doing it right. No one stepped off the page to make the movements come alive for me. A couple of years passed and I took a workshop. That helped, but the experience was only for the day. When I got home, I found that I couldn't remember all the instructions. Nor could I watch the teacher again. Eventually, I attended massage school to become a professional therapist and I went on to teach others how to massage.

Years later, I realized there was a need for a way to bring massage to more people in a non-classroom setting. For the first time in history we have the technology to learn an ancient art in a new way. That's why I was delighted when producer Steve Adams and Shari Belafonte asked me to work with them and James Heartland on the "Massage For Health" video. Finally, I can share—through movements on the screen and words in this handbook—the massage experience. Massage has opened many doors for me—getting to know the body and the language of touch, understanding myself and my relations with others, reaching into my heart and finding compassion, becoming sensitive to another's pain and having a way to help relieve it. It has opened doors to people, places, and situations I could never have imagined possible.

I invite you to open the first door by learning massage. Massage will do the rest. It will help you relax and combat stress, add pleasure to your relationships, improve your athletic activity, help you sleep restfully, enhance your sensuality and much more. As you feel better, you'll look better too. You'll also be able to communicate non-verbally with greater sensitivity as you develop an inner awareness, an intuitive capacity through your hands.

I wish I'd had "Massage For Health" when I first embarked on my massage odyssey. I would have been able to give a better massage a lot sooner. Enjoy.

MASSACE,
UNIVERSAL AND TIMELESS

For thousands of years, massage has been effectively used throughout the world. It has been practiced not only by massage professionals, but also by doctors, midwives, sports trainers, religious shamans, and teachers of dance and martial arts.

Nearly two decades of travel and study have shown me how prevalent and appreciated massage is, particularly in non-Western cultures. Healers frequently use massage to help members of their community recover from sundry ailments. The people themselves also massage each other to get over the physical exertion of work and sports. It's a dynamic way to strengthen intimate bonds with their loved ones, young and old. They massage children to grow healthy and strong and massage the elderly to ease their aches and pains and stem the tide of loneliness. Yet massage plays more than an obviously therapeutic role. It's also a gesture of hospitality extended to visitors, a sign of respect and gratitude, and a sensual prelude to lovemaking.

Asia, more than any other continent, demonstrates that — contrary to what some people believe — massage is not a luxury limited to the wealthy. It is a commonly accepted practice available for everyone's benefit. In a Nepalese courtyard I watched a mother massaging her baby in the warmth of the winter sun. As I alighted from a ferry to Koh Samui, an island off the east coast of Thailand, I saw men publicly massaged in a wooden pavilion at the water's edge.

Massage has played its part in America too. North American Indians, Mexicans, and other ethnic groups have used it in childbirth, healing ceremonies, and for the treatment of psychological disorders. In the late 1800s and early 1900s, many medical doctors here (and in Europe) continued a tradition begun by ancient Greek and Roman physicians. They routinely prescribed massage — some even did massage themselves — for anything from insomnia to paralysis. For many decades into the twentieth century, massage was included in a nurse's training. It was also the foundation on which the field of physical therapy was established in World War I. But as the pressure of time and the high cost of medical attention increased, health professionals opted for technological advances instead of hands-on work. Massage *nearly* became a forgotten healing art in the United States.

Today, massage is once again being acknowledged as a universal tool of healing, pleasure, and communication. It's a timely revival. For as we question why our modern lifestyle in the richest country in the world is not leading to the peace and contentment we anticipated, we're also exploring how else we can find happiness and satisfaction. We're discovering that it's where we least expected it—in ourselves and the people we share our lives with.

People living in traditional cultures consistently maintain face-to-face relations in their daily interactions with others. But we live in a society that continues to replace direct human contact with impersonal time-saving equipment. We drive up to a box to order our food from a disembodied voice. We stand at a faceless window teller to make a bank deposit. More and more technology and a faster pace of living disconnect us not only from one another, but also from ourselves. Although surrounded by people, we may feel isolated. We can break down these invisible barriers and truly get back in touch by actually touching.

Many of us are also frustrated and dissatisfied with a health care system that is often indifferent, even dehumanizing. We want to be considered as more than a physical body to be repaired. We also have psychological and spiritual needs that machines and medication don't address. But touch does. Massage reaches all aspects of our being because it's not just physical therapy. Through our hands we share what is in our hearts. While medical technology and pharmaceuticals serve their purpose, they can't ever convey the concern we feel through the touch of someone who cares about our well-being.

Nor do drugs and alcohol answer our deeper needs. In fact, their serious side effects compound the stress we try to reduce by using them. In our need for alternatives to energize us or calm us down, more and more people, like you, are realizing that we have the basic source of healing and pleasure right at our fingertips.

What could be more basic than the simple act of touching? Instinctively we use our hands to help ourselves and each other. Think of how often you immediately rub the part of your body that you've just hurt. Consider, too, the wave of immense pleasure you feel when your partner caresses you.

Our passion for high-performance sports, our commitment to fitness and our need to combat stress have also renewed enthusiasm for massage. But you don't have to be Olympic athletes Mary Decker Slaney or Edwin Moses to include massage in your exercise regimen. Nor do you have to be Chrysler Corporation's Lee Iacocca to use it in stress reduction. Massage is for everyone—executives and housewives, marathon competitors and weekend tennis players, 8-month-old babies and 75-year-old grandmothers.

And, you don't have to wait until you're really hurting to justify having a massage. Massage is an invaluable tool in preventive care. It can make you more aware of critical bodily cues so that you take a break before you break down.

By bringing massage into your life, you're taking a positive step for your health. You're learning to understand the language of your own body. You're using touch to say "yes" to relaxation and pleasure and "no" to tension and pain.

OUR SENSE OF TOUCH

Like plants that need rain and sunshine to grow, we need to be nourished by touch. As babies, we can't survive without it. Infants who are not held have been known to die of "marasmus," a wasting away. In a series of experiments more than twenty years ago, psychologist Harry Harlow showed that touch can be even more critical than food. When offered a bare wire surrogate "mother" with a nipple providing milk and a soft, cloth-covered "mother" with no milk, baby monkeys gave up food for physicial contact.

Touch begins in the womb. Every movement a pregnant woman makes massages and stimulates the child inside her. Labor contractions actually provide a vital massage which helps the baby to start breathing and helps its blood to circulate. After birth touch helps keep the nervous system growing and that enables us to develop our motor skills.

This essential physical closeness at the beginning of our lives is also a source of emotional nourishment. Reassuring touch gives us a sense of security and strength with which to meet the new world around us, for our entire awakening is experienced through the body. Later, when we're upset as adults, a comforting touch can soothe us as much as it did when we were held and stroked as children. It may be why touch is so integral to our health and happiness long after childhood and into old age, which so often is a time of loneliness. And it may be why massage became the first healing art. Studies indicate that even stroking a pet can lower your own blood pressure.

Touch is unique among our senses. What we touch touches us; what touches us is also touched by us. But what we see or hear is unaffected by our eyes and ears. Physical contact helps us comprehend something in a way that seeing alone does not. Touch gives us another sense—in-sight—as though we could see with our hands, even our whole body. Taught to look with our eyes and know with our intellect, we forget how much more we can understand through inner awareness. In places like Japan and Indonesia, blind people have traditionally been trained in the art of massage. It is believed that their sense of touch is greater because they lack the sense of sight.

Massage helps us to redress the imbalance between our left brain, which emphasizes logical, rational thought, and our right brain, which focuses on our intuitive capacity. As one psychologist has suggested, it's time to let go of our mind and come to our senses.

HOW MASSAGE WORKS

The miracle of touch and massage lies in the skin. Surprisingly, it's the largest organ in the body and as important as the brain, heart, and lungs in keeping us alive. In an area the size of a quarter, the skin contains more than 3 million cells, 100 sweat glands, 50 nerve endings and 3 feet of blood vessels. But massage is not just skin deep.

As the embryo grows, its outermost cells become the skin, hair, nails, and teeth; and the sense organs of touch, hearing, taste, vision and smell, which make us aware of what is going on externally. From the underside of this layer of cells comes the central nervous system (the brain and spinal cord), which informs us of what is going on internally. This connection between what we feel on the outside and what we feel on the inside makes the skin a kind of switchboard for incoming and outgoing messages.

The pressure we apply in massage also affects what's beneath the skin. We loosen up muscles that are tight from exercise and tension. We help blood and lymph circulate so that all parts of the body can receive essential nutrients like oxygen, get rid of waste products, and defend against disease. We stimulate sensory receptors that relay signals to our body systems, telling them to relax or gear up. Some doctors have suggested that massage may even trigger the release of endorphins, the body's natural opiates that lead to euphoric feelings and pain relief.

Massage works so well because we have billions of sensory receptors throughout our bodies. Our hands alone contain approximately one and a half million, with the greatest concentration in our fingertips. That's why there's no substitute for human touch. Massage machines can never know what you feel through your own hands.

Try for youself. Place your hands on a part of your partner's body. Then close your eyes and take a few minutes to explore how it feels. Is it soft and smooth or hard and knotted? Is it warm or cold? Does the tissue contract in response to your touch or does it relax? The Hawaiians taught healing in this way. Blindfolded, a student would learn to "see" with her fingers so that later she could know the nature of a person's discomfort merely by feeling him. By paying attention to the particular sensations you feel while giving a massage, eventually you will become skillful in distinguishing what the body is saying.

Just as massage is more than skin deep, it's also more than physiology. A loving touch can spark the inner will to become well, for it sends a message of healing or health, words which originally meant whole and unhurt. That message can help activate the healing potential we all possess in order to harmonize the energies of our mind, body and spirit. Ultimately, healing is an act of kindness, helping someone to feel better physicially and emotionally through the communication of wholeness.

DIFFERENT TOUCH THERAPIES

A message of healing or wholeness can be communicated through a variety of body-oriented therapies. The French word "massage" originally referred to kneading, but over the centuries it has evolved as a generic term that includes many kinds of body manipulations performed in countries around the world. Although the systems that are popular today— Shiatsu, Swedish, Rolfing, Reflexology, and Polarity, to name only a few—approach healing through different theories and techniques, they all aim to relieve discomfort and restore balance through touch.

When we talk about massage, we generally mean Swedish or *Swedish/Easlen* style, the most well-known form of Western massage today and the one you learn in "Massage For Health." Many people prefer it because while you're enjoying thereapeutic benefits, the gliding movements on lubricated skin also result in a pleasurable sensual experience.

Based on Western anatomy and physiology, Swedish massage works directly with the body's structure. It combines systematic stroking, rubbing, kneading, pressing and vibrating of the soft tissues, with stretching and joint rotation. These manipulations relax muscles and relieve soreness, stimulate blood and lymph circulation, calm the nervous system, reduce swelling and adhesions, and promote a feeling of well-being. For athletic people there's the added benefit of flushing out the chemical by-products of exercise.

Developed by Peter Ling of Sweden in the nineteenth century, Swedish massage was later modified in California during the 1960s and '70s. Practitioners at the Esalen Institute felt that massage should be a more soothing experience and deal with more than the receiver's physical state. By using greater sensitivity and your own intuition, you can more skillfully perceive the receiver's needs and adapt the massage accordingly.

A full body Swedish massage is generally given on a specially designed table, although many people are able to work effectively on the floor as well. The receiver is at least partially undressed so that oil can be used to lubricate the skin for smoother movements.

Oriental massage approaches the body through a different philosophy. By unblocking and stimulating circulation of the life force, called *chi* or *ki*, so that it flows freely along energy pathways called meridians, you help prevent illness and allow the body to heal itself. In Shiatsu, acupressure, Do-In, and Jin Shin Do, you use your fingers, hands, elbows, even feet and knees to apply pressure on tiny prescribed points along 14 meridians. While acupressure confines itself to acupuncture points, the other three methods also incorporate stretching. Oriental massage is commonly done on the floor and can be given directly through the receiver's clothing.

Other forms of bodywork include reflexology, or zone therapy, sports massage and Rolfing. Reflexology is based on the theory that pressure applied to various points on the feet or hands relieves symptoms in corresponding organs and glands. Sports massage integrates Swedish movements with pressure-point techniques to prevent injury, improve athletic performance, and aid recovery. Special attention is paid to the areas of the body most stressed by the particular sport. Rolfing or Structural Integration strives to remove structural imbalances and align the body through very deep massage of the fascia, connective tissue which surrounds every muscle. Still other systems, like Polarity, Feldenkrais and Tragering, are based on the stimulation of electrochemical and neuro-muscular reflexes.

Although the various body therapies use different techniques, a good Swedish massage actually unites all of them. Although we don't intentionally massage acupuncture points, the pressure we apply all over the body reaches many of them. When we relieve muscular tension, we also relax emotional tension and unblock energy. And because there are billions of sensory receptors located throughout the body, massage has many reflexive effects on digestion, excretion, hormonal secretion, etc.

Some massage therapists specialize in one or another of the bodywork systems. Others are eclectic, combining several to suit the varied needs of their clients. With "Massage For Health" you'll be building a foundation to which you can add other techniques in the future.

CAUTION

Although massage has been used to treat all kinds of ailments, it is not a panacea and it is not a substitute for sound medical advice. The information presented here does not replace professional medical attention. Be sure to check with your doctor to find out whether you have any conditions which massage might aggravate, such as a fracture, dislocation or severe sprain. Don't massage if there is acute infection or inflammation, fever, skin disease and hemorrhaging, or if there are large hernias, tumors, burns and abscesses. Avoid massage in such cardiovascular problems as advanced arteriosclerosis, aneurysms, severe varicose veins, thrombosis and acute phlebitis.

GETTING READY

MENTAL AND PHYSICAL PREPARATION

Massage is a unique experience. I like to think of it as a special date, a commitment to meaningful contact. Whether I give or receive a massage, there are some basic ways I prepare myself in order to make it an enjoyable and memorable time. Before making any physical arrangements, it's important to be in the right frame of mind first. If you've ever felt hesitant about massage, remember that you're not alone. Even if you're not new to the massage experience, consider the following in preparing yourself mentally. You'll see what a difference it can make.

DON'T WAIT

So many people I've massaged for their first time invariably exclaim afterward, "I can't believe I waited so long to do this." Too often we postpone special experiences because we want to have things perfect first. But just as you don't have to own fancy gear in order to be in the great outdoors, you don't have to use elaborate equipment in order to massage. For now, all you really need is your hands, a caring attitude, and sensitivity. Later, you might decide to buy or build a massage table, or even add a hot tub or sauna to your home.

LET GO OF FEARS

Many of us lacked positive touching when we were growing up and may be inhibited about touch in general, even afraid that it implies sex. Take heart. Any time we reach out to share with someone else, we're taking a risk, but the rewards are usually worth it. Whether you're giving or receiving a massage, you may feel safer at first with massage of the hands, feet or head. Later, move on to larger areas, such as the back or legs. As you get used to the pleasurable sensations of massage, gradually you'll become very comfortable with both touching and being touched.

Part of preparing for a massage is checking your energy level and feelings. Are you too tired or sick to do a massage? Don't push yourself to give what you haven't got. Arrange to do the massage another time. Is there unfinished business between you and your partner? If either of you is angry about something, resolve what you can now and close the door on the rest. It is important to have open communication so you both fully enjoy the massage, but if you put off massage until you've cleared up all your problems, you'll never get to it.

When checking your feelings, be honest with yourself. Are you using massage as another arena in which to perform? *Don't pressure yourself.* Massage is not a race in which you're competing with other athletes. Neither is it a sale you have to make to rack up commissions. Massage is an experience to approach gently—with love, compassion, and respect—not only for the person you massage, but also for yourself. So relax and be patient while you're learning. You're not going to ruin the whole massage if you botch a stroke.

Being honest also means being realistic about what you can do. Let go of inflated expectations, especially at the beginning. With practice your confidence and competence will grow. However, keep in mind that your partner's body is not a machine and you're not a technician who is going to repair it. Nor is massage a cure-all. Don't be disappointed if you don't see spectacular results. Although one massage can make a big difference in how someone feels, massage is more effective when repeated regularly. It's also more effective if you avoid working deeply at first. Without the necessary skill, you're more likely to give pain than relief. And, if your partner drifts off during the massage, don't be concerned. Massage works its magic even if she falls asleep.

Agreeing with your partner on some guidelines before you get started will help you avoid some awkward moments. Find out if there is any part of your partner's body he doesn't want you to touch. Determine whether you have enough time for a complete massage. *A partial massage can be just as relaxing and as much fun.* Especially when you first start practicing, you'll probably deal with only one area at a time, incorporating others as you learn them. This way you'll not only increase your self-confidence and skill, you'll also increase your strength so you can do a whole body massage without tiring.

With these understandings in mind, you're ready to go to the physical preparation .

In my travels, I've been surprised by how public massage is in many countries. You can see it at a park, on a rooftop, or even in the street. Just outside the gates of the Taj Mahal I watched a group of people standing around a masseur and the man he worked on, talking freely with both of them and with each other. But in the West, massage is generally a quiet, private experience in order to promote a sense of caring intimacy and a deep state of relaxation. In that state, all your senses are heightened. That's why it's important to *create a comfortable environment* where you won't be interrupted.

AVOID DISTRACTIONS

Ringing telephones, noisy appliances, strong odors, and restless pets are not conducive to relaxation. Try to pick a time when no one else will be around. If you can, arrange for children to stay with their friends or neighbors for a while. (Save massage with your kids for another time.) Remember to unplug your phone or put your answering machine on.

ADJUST THE TEMPERATURE

Whichever room you use, *make sure it's warm enough for your partner,* even if it means it will be too warm for you. (You can keep a towel handy in case you perspire heavily.) You know what it feels like to be cold: you can't relax because your muscles stay contracted. An electric blanket can prevent chilling, particularly during the winter months. Place it underneath a sheet ahead of time so that when the person lies down, the area is already warm. Then turn down the blanket setting for the massage. A good alternative is to keep extra sheets or blankets handy.

If you live in a hot climate or if it's summertime, you might want to turn on a fan. Or, for a lovely change, go outdoors. Find a soft, but level place in the shade, just so long as insects aren't a problem.

APPEAL TO ALL THE SENSES

Tone down the lighting. It's hard to relax under bright lights even with closed eyes. Also check that sunlight isn't shining directly onto your partner's face. If you want to use music to set a mood or muffle other sounds, like traffic and humming refrigerators, keep it soft. Stay away from anything that has such a distinct beat you find yourself following it instead of your own rhythm. Add a light fragrance to the room with flowers or incense. Set the mood according to the situation you're in; romantic candlelight may not always be appropriate.

These simple touches make the difference between a sensual massage experience and the clinical kind you might get in a hospital. But that doesn't mean you can skip what's important in a medical setting.

BE CLEAN

No one likes to lie down on dirty floors and dirty linen, so be sure the space and the things you use are clean. Don't forget personal hygiene either. Before a massage, it's fun and relaxing to take a shower, bath, hot tub or sauna, alone or together. It will help get both of you in the mood and take care of most body odors. If you're the receiver and your skin is gritty or sandy because you've been outdoors, washing up will keep the massage from feeling rough. If you're the giver and your partner has an unpleasant odor, cover the problem area with a towel. Most people are unaware of how they smell. In some cases, an offensive odor may be the result of diet or poor health. Talk it over sensitively.

Wash your hands before giving the massage and make sure your fingernails are not long and ragged. You don't want to leave your mark on anyone. Remember to wash your hands again right after the massage.

LESS IS BETTER

Wear as little clothing as possible and make sure it's loose so you can move about freely. A full body oil massage is best done on a person who is nude, but if your partner feels more comfortable wearing a bathing suit or underwear, respect her decision.

Remove your own and your partner's jewelry. It interferes with stroking smoothly. It also feels cold to the touch and can scratch the skin.

If your partner is wearing contact lenses, ask him to remove them for greater relaxation. Otherwise, merely avoid direct pressure on the eyes when you massage the face.

In preparing for a massage, you may not always be able to create the "ideal" setting. If your friend has just come back from a long run or bike ride, you're outside, and there's no shower, pad or blanket, work with what you have. *Improvise rather than avoid massage just because you don't have perfect conditions.* What's more important is the atmosphere you create with your own attitude and ingenuity.

ACCESSORIES

Working on the floor is a good beginning. Although using a massage table affords you greater mobility and flexibility and less strain, you may want to wait until later to invest in one.

For now, lay down a pad or several blankets (unless you have plush carpeting) and cover them with a sheet or large towel to avoid possible oil stains. Since you'll be on your knees a lot, make sure there's enough padding for you too as you work your way around your partner's body.

Don't use a bed unless it's a hard platform with a foam pad or futon. On regular beds, you can't apply enough pressure to keep the person from sinking into the mattress.

Whatever you massage on, move carefully so that you don't incur problems in your own body, especially your back.

As you massage, keep checking your position. Does it allow you to move fluidly, with strength, or are you getting tense and tired? Take a moment to adjust your posture. If you're relaxed, then the massage you give will be relaxing.

Since comfort is the keynote, *keep pillows, rolled up towels or blankets around to provide extra support and padding.* People with low back problems appreciate a pillow under their knees to ease the arch that's accentuated when they're lying on their back. For the same reason, they also like one under their abdomen when they're face down. A pillow under the ankles helps the feet to relax.

Whatever lubricant you use, make sure you have enough so you don't run out in the middle of the massage. For convenience, you might want to have some at either end of the body.

LUBRICANTS

When giving a whole body massage, it's important to lubricate the skin. It reduces friction, pinching, and pulling of body hair. How much of a lubricant you use depends on your partner's skin. Dry skin and hairy areas absorb more and may require reapplication. Oily skin needs only a light film to make your movements smooth and even, rather than jerky.

There are several kinds of lubricants, each with different benefits and drawbacks. Oil is slippery and takes longer to absorb. It's an easier base for blending in concentrated essential oils, such as eucalpytus, peppermint and cinnamon, which help create more heat in the muscles to relieve aches. Vegetable oils can leave stains, so don't use your best sheets. Mineral oil is clear, odorless, and does not stain, but because it is a derivative of petroleum, it is not recommended for body use.

For people who do not enjoy oil on their skin, lotion is soothing, but it contains alcohol, which evaporates quickly and leaves a cooling sensation. That means you have to keep reapplying the lotion in order to massage smoothly. If oil alone seems too greasy, pour a little lotion and a little oil into your palm and mix them together. If someone is allergic to both oil and lotion, try powder.

You can purchase already bottled massage oil or prepare it yourself by blending several oils together or using only one kind. Sunflower and safflower are fairly light and neutral while olive oil is heavier and has a more noticeable smell. Coconut oil is popular in tropical climates, like southern

India and the Pacific Islands. Or try sesame, peanut, avocado, almond or apricot kernel oil. Add a few drops of extract like vanilla, lemon or almond to give the oil a pleasant fragrance, but don't overpower it with a strong perfume.

If you live in a cold climate, it's good to warm the oil ahead of time. You can place the plastic bottle in a container of hot water instead of heating it up on the stove. But even when the oil is warm, don't pour it directly onto the person's skin or let it accidentally drip. Put a little oil in one palm and then rub your hands together, warming the oil some more before applying it. Instead of oiling the whole body all at once, lubricate only the area you'll be working on immediately so that it doesn't dry out.

If you use just enough oil to glide your hands across the body, the skin will absorb it and you won't have to rub off excess oil with a towel. If you apply too much oil, you'll have difficulty maintaining contact. Remember not to oil your hands before massaging the head. Also, most people have enough oil in their face to massage without a lubricant.

Have a wet washcloth and dry towel available when the massage is over. Use it to remove oil from your partner's feet to avoid stains once he gets up and walks around. Many people like to keep the massage oil on their body as a moisturizer, but if your partner doesn't like it, just wipe it off.

All these details may seem like a lot to remember at first, but don't worry. As you practice massage, they'll become second nature to you.

CENTERING

In creating an environment that is conducive to total relaxation, you want to have quiet, comfort, and no interruptions or distractions. But even more important is the atmosphere you establish with your own state of mind, so take a few moments to center yourself in the way that works best for you or follow the instructions in the section on centering and breath. And keep the following in mind.

STAY CENTERED
Once you start the massage, if your mind races, don't follow it. When you're busy thinking about what was and what might be, you lose the opportunity to experience what is happening in the present. Take a deep breath and refocus on the massage.

AVOID UNNECESSARY TALKING
After your initial discussion, keep your words to a minimum during the massage. Both of you need to put your full attention on it. Try to communicate with your touch instead of your voice as much as possible.

BE OPEN TO FEEDBACK AND CHANGES

Being quiet is important during a massage, but so is vital feedback. If you get so involved in the massage that you don't want to stop, check with your partner to see if it's okay to go past the time agreed on. When you receive a massage, don't be shy about letting him know how you feel. If his strokes are too intense, if some parts of your body are especially sensitive or if you have an injury, let him know. Don't grin and bear the pain. The same is true if you have to go to the bathroom. It's okay to interrupt the massage in order to take care of your needs. And if you want more detail in a particular area, don't hesitate to ask for a little extra. These kinds of communications help avoid resentment towards your partner and disappointment in the massage he gave you. If you really like the massage you're getting, words or sounds of enjoyment will instill more confidence in him.

BE SENSITIVE

Many people aren't satisfied with their body as it is. They think they're too fat or too thin; they'd like a slimmer waist or broader shoulders. Conveying a non-judgmental attitude will enable others to relax more. *Touch lovingly*, sensitively. Expressing something positive about the person's body helps too: "you have a nice strong back" or "your hands are graceful."

STAY COOL

Massage is a sensual experience. Sometimes it indirectly results in sexual arousal. Such reactions are natural, but you don't need to concentrate on them, for they arise and then pass away. And, you don't have to do anything about them unless you've both already planned to.

MEDITATION

With the right attitude and preparation, massage can be a dynamic meditation—an expression of quiet concentration *and* physical movement that you can share with others, instead of only yourself. When you still your mind, you can focus or center your energy so that you massage more sensitively, more intuitively. *Simply watching your breath is a gateway into a deeper state of awareness that allows you to open to that intuitive source within.*

When we consciously pay attention to our breath, we can use it to help ourselves relax and enable our body to live in optimal health. It's a very basic process. As we inhale, oxygen rushes in to nourish every cell in the body. As we exhale, carbon dioxide rushes out. When we breathe shallowly, our lungs and heart have to work harder to supply oxygen to the whole body so that it can continuously heal itself.

Getting in touch with your breath is an easy way to make contact with yourself before you make contact with your partner. Here is a simple exercise for doing that.

🌱 Sit comfortably in a straight-backed chair or cross-legged on the floor. Without straining, keep your spine erect and let your hands rest loosely on your thighs. Close your eyes and focus on your abdomen. As you inhale, feel it expand. As you exhale, feel it sink back in again. Don't try to make your breath shorter or longer, faster or slower. Just sense the rhythm as it is. Also, don't force yourself to take the next breath, but wait until it's ready to come on its own. As you become more aware of your breath, you'll notice a natural pause after each exhalation.

🌱 To help focus your attention even more, note "rising" as your belly expands on an in-breath and "falling" as it contracts on an out-breath. If your attention wanders— maybe you feel your rib cage enlarging too—don't change how you're breathing, just go back to observing the "rising" and "falling" of your belly.

By gathering your energy into one area, it will be stronger, more concentrated for you to work with during the massage. The more balanced you become, the more you'll be able to experience the massage in the present moment, without thinking back to the past or looking ahead to the future. The more present you are, the more you'll be able to hear what your partner's body communicates to you and to know what to communicate back to it through your touch.

CENTERING TOGETHER

For even greater harmony in the massage, here's an exercise you can both do to get centered together.

🌱 Sit back to back so that you're in close contact, supporting one another equally. Follow the directions for the first breath exercise. For the moment, forget about your partner and just watch your own breath. Once you're in tune with your rhythm of breathing, bring your partner's rhythm into focus too. Gradually, without trying to quickly change anything, let your breath synchronize with his. If you get out of tune, slowly ease back into it. Spend about five minutes breathing together.

STAYING FOCUSED

If you find that your mind wanders, once you start the massage, don't follow it. When you're busy thinking about what was and what might be, you lose the opportunity to feel what is happening in the present. Take a deep breath and refocus. Staying focused during the massage is important in making it a meaningful and effective experience. Here are several ways you can do that.

As the giver:

🌿 When you first make contact with your partner, let your hands rest lightly on his upper back and slowly match your breath pattern with his. Breathing in unison will help you to be more in tune with the needs of your partner.

🌿 While giving the massage, check that you're neither holding your breath and stiffening up nor breathing so quickly that you're racing through the movements. In order for your touch to bring about relaxation in the person you massage, you need to be relaxed too.

🌿 Another way to avoid tensing up during the massage is by centering on your partner's body and, at the same time, imagining that your strokes are relaxing that part of your body too.

🌿 Tuning into your breath will also help you to work more easily. It's just a matter of coordinating it with your movements. For example, *remember to exhale when you move your body forward in a stroke and to inhale as you lean back on the return stroke.* This will enable you to be stronger without straining your own back. Don't worry about perfect timing all at once. With practice, you'll find that synchronizing your breath with the massage strokes and your body movements will become effortless, as you develop a rhythm that turns your massage into a healing dance.

As the receiver:

🌿 When you first lie down and your partner has made contact with you, take several deep breaths. On an in-breath, imagine fresh energy and relaxation entering through your feet and flowing all the way to your head. On an out-breath, feel all the tension drain right out your feet. With each breath, notice how you sink deeper into the floor or table.

🌿 Once the massage begins, you can use your breath to help release stress from your body. As you relax, you become more aware of where you hold tension. When your partner reaches a particularly tight place, consciously exhale as he applies pressure; inhale as he lightens his touch. As he harmonizes his pressure with your breath, you'll be working together to loosen contracted muscles. You can also mentally massage the area by visualizing it as a knot

21

you untie or steel cables that you separate (or whatever image works for you). *By massaging internally with your breath and your mind, you're assisting your partner to better help you.* But be sure that you don't try to physically help him by lifting your own limbs or head. You'll get the most out of the massage by completely letting go and allowing yourself to totally receive.

Whether you're the giver or receiver, remember that massage is not a mechanical manipulation. Touch is a constant exchange of non-verbal messages flowing through the hands. You're both exploring who the other person is and simultaneously communicating about your discoveries. By staying focused, in a meditative state, you'll be better able to let your intuition guide you in the process of exploration, discovery, and communication.

MASSAGE

USING YOUR HANDS

Hands...we use them for a thousand and one tasks every day. But how well do we know them? Take a few moments to get acquainted with your hands. It will help your massage immeasurably.

With one hand, explore the different parts of your other hand. Feel where it is soft and fleshy, hard and bony, flat or sharp, smooth or rough. Change hands and repeat.

Then, using those different parts—the palm, heel and side of your hands, the fingers, thumbs, and knuckles—experiment with how each one feels as you continue the exploration on your arm or leg. As you move up and down your limb, notice how some parts of your hands are more suited than others for a particular place. For example, it's easier and more effective to use your thumb and fingers rather than your palm when massaging around the elbow and wrist joints. Notice, too, the difference between rubbing with the tips of your fingers or thumbs and using the fleshy pads, even when you don't have long nails. You'll be able to better control your pressure and avoid sharpness by massaging with the pads. You'll also find it easier to keep your hands relaxed.

Relaxed hands are the key to massaging firmly but gently. They're more flexible, better able to bend, curve and mold to the contours of the body. Tense hands feel hard and can't convey a message of relaxation. Relaxed hands are like a stream that flows over and around the branches and rocks in its path. When your hands are relaxed, the fingers stay together and increase the area of contact. If you're massaging with only your thumb, the rest of your hand will lightly touch the body rather than stick stiffly into the air.

To start off your massage with relaxed hands, get into the habit of loosely shaking them. Standing up or leaning forward in your seat, imagine that your arms are wet noodles, limp and dangling, as you shake out any tension. Be sure your wrists are floppy or your hands will tense up even more. If you find yourself stiffening up during the massage, pause to shake out again. It's better to stop for a moment than to keep massaging with tense hands. Also, when your hands are relaxed, you're more sensitive and less likely to hurt anyone. Your movements will be smoother and steadier. Maintaining an even tempo in your strokes makes for a more enjoyable massage.

Staying relaxed can help you with pressure too. If you're unsure about how much pressure to use, practice on yourself first, then on your partner, and ask him for feedback. Most people are not built like China dolls. Still, applying pressure gradually is the least intrusive way of penetrating stiff muscles and communicating to them to let go. If your touch is too deep too soon, your partner will tense up to resist the pressure. So, *start lightly, slowly increase your pressure, then lighten up again as you finish the stroke.*

If you think your hands aren't strong enough to apply good pressure, don't let that inhibit you. The more you massage, the stronger your hands will become. However, the greatest strength comes not from your hands themselves, but from putting your body weight behind the stroke. Although you need to focus on what your hands are doing, you also need to be aware of the rest of your body. Rocking back and forth or side to side, depending on the position you're in, will enable you to build a steady, even rhythm and keep you from getting tired. When you use your whole body, not just your hands, you will find that massage can be a healing dance for you and your partner.

STROKES

To establish a foundation in Swedish massage, you need several basic building blocks or strokes. Each one serves a different but important purpose in making the massage feel good and be effective. You use the same ones over and over again, varying them according to the part of the body you're massaging. As you grow in confidence and skill, you'll find yourself becoming more creative with the fundamental strokes, the way an artist combines primary colors to achieve an unlimited range of hues in painting a picture.

EFFLEURAGE/STROKING

Effleurage or stroking can feel like water gliding and rippling over the body. It's a good way to begin and complete any large area, like the back, legs or arms. Use it to smoothe on oil and get acquainted with the condition of the muscles. By starting light and gradually increasing your pressure, you can warm up the muscles for deeper work. Repeated rhythmically, stroking can have a lulling or hypnotic effect that leads to relaxation. By pressing firmly in the direction of the heart, you can assist the return flow of blood and lymph. You can stroke long, up and down the body, or wide, across the body, or in broad circles. To make your movements fluid and soothing, stroke with the entire flat surface of the palms (fingers or arms) and keep your fingers together. Used as a connecting stroke, effleurage will help you make a smooth transition from one area to the next and integrate all parts of the body at the very end. Like gentle clouds, let strokes float onto the body when you first start and float away as you finish.

PETRISSAGE/KNEADING

Kneading often follows deep stroking to further relax the muscles, aid circulation of blood and lymph, and mobilize metabolic by-products for faster recovery from fatigue. As in kneading dough, you alternate your hands and rhymthically pick up and squeeze a fleshy area of the body, such as the buttocks, thighs, or calves. You apply pressure, then release, progressing through the area as you repeat the grasping and compressing. Used during rehabilitation, these movements help keep muscles supple and elastic and minimize the formation of fibrous tissue and adhesions that generally result from injury.

FRICTION

Friction movements tend to be small, firm, and circular. After stroking or kneading, you use them to penetrate more deeply and also work around the joints. By applying pressure with a fingerpad, thumb, fist or heel of your hand in a round motion or across the muscles (cross-fiber friction), you can help break up knots and adhesions and spread muscle fibers in a limited area, such as the Achilles tendon. The benefits of friction are increased if you follow it with more stroking and kneading.

TAPOTEMENT/PERCUSSION

Like kneading, percussion calls for alternating the hands, only this time in a series of quick, short, rhythmic move-

ments. Depending on the area stimulated, you use the outer
border of your hand and relaxed fingers (hacking), loosely
clenched fists (pummeling or pounding), or cupped hands
(cupping) to strike the muscles without bruising them. Along
with plucking or pinching, these percussive strokes stimulate
muscles, nerves, and circulation and help tone the skin.

VIBRATION

Gently shaking or jostling muscles helps loosen them,
especially when they're too sore for deep strokes. You can
vibrate a small area with the palm of your hand or fingers or
shake an entire leg or arm. If the receiver has difficulty letting
go, vibration can help break the holding pattern and relax
the area while also invigorating it.

STRETCHING AND JOINT ROTATION

Gentle rotation of joints through their range of motion
helps improve flexibility. Be careful to take a joint only as far as
it will go and be sure you lift without any physical help from
the receiver. Slow stretching coordinated with the breath
can also help loosen tight muscles and increase flexibility.

MASSAGE SEQUENCE

When learning massage, it's useful at the beginning to follow a specific pattern of moving from one part of the body
to another. Memorizing the sequence eliminates having to
think about what to do next and allows you to concentrate
more on how you're massaging. There are other good reasons
to follow the order taught in "Massage For Health"—they're
explained in the introduction to each body area. Once you
improve your skill and build your confidence, you can create
your own order to suit each individual massage you give. It's
like playing jazz: once you know the composition, you can
go off and improvise to your heart's content.

We start with the back, move down to the back of the legs,
go to the front of the legs, the abdomen and chest, arms, and
finish with head/face. *Each time you approach a part of the
body, you begin by applying oil (except on the head/face) only
to the area you'll be massaging.* Otherwise, the oil could be
absorbed before you reach that section and your partner
could cool off.

*Stroke lightly at first, progressively going deeper, then finishing
with light strokes again.* Both at the beginning and at the end,
be sure to cover the whole area with some long movements.
Your initial strokes serve as an introduction, letting your partner know where you'll be massaging next. Your final strokes
will give him a sense of completion. After you've massaged
both the upper and lower parts of the front or back, you can

WHOLE BODY ~~~~~~~~~~~~~~
MASSAGE SEQUENCE
~~~~~~~~~~~~~~~~~~~~~~~~~~~~~~

I. *THE BACK* is a wonderful place to start because almost everyone feels safe getting a "backrub." As the largest, flat-test area of the body, the back is an excellent classroom for learning the strokes that you'll apply on other parts of the body. If you're unable to do a full-body massage, working on the back alone can give a sense of deep release because of tension most people hold there. Begin with light pressure and increase gradually. *Do not massage directly on the spine.*

1. Making Contact.
2. Oiling and Effleurage.
3. Thumb Stroking.
4. Thumb Friction Circles.
5. Forearm Effleurage.
6. Shoulder Kneading.
7. Shoulder Blade Vibration.
8. Side Kneading.
9. Forearm Pulling.
10. Palm Circles.
11. Forearm Stretch.

II. *THE LEGS AND FEET* transports us all day long from place to place, whether we're simply walking or engaging in sports. Massage helps prepare them for exercise by bringing more oxygen to the muscles. The back of the legs is a great place to knead out metabolic by-products which cause soreness and fatigue after physical activity. *Do not press hard behind the knee.*

1. Effleurage & Oiling.
2. V-Effleurage.
3. Chain of V-Effleurages.
4. Kneading.
5. V-Effleurage.
6. Fist Friction Circles.
7. V-Effleurage.
8. Calf Shake.
9. Heel-To-Buttock Stretch.
10. Ankle Rotation and Twist.
11. Effleurage and Oil Feet.
12. Small Friction Circles.
13. Heel of Hand Circles.
14. Thumb Circles.
15. Hand Effleurage.
16. Percussion.
17. Connecting Stroke.
18. Spinal Finger Walk.

III. *THE FRONT OF LEGS AND FEET.*

1. Pillow Positioning.
2. Effleurage and Oiling.
3. Kneading.
4. Thigh Cross Stroke.
5. Effleurage.
6. Foot Effleurage.
7. Foot Knead.
8. Heel Squeeze.
9. Toe Knead.
10. Foot Spread.
11. Forearm Friction Circles.
12. Thigh Roll.
13. Knee-to-Chest Stretch.
14. Knee Rotation.
15. Pull and Shake.
16. Rocking & Connecting.

IV. *THE FRONT OF THE BODY* is a vulnerable place for most people. Approach it with great sensitivity and respect. Massaging the chest helps relax the muscles around the ribs so we can expand our capacity to breathe. Because some people feel ticklish in the ribs, make your strokes firm and slow. If your partner has a lower back problem, put a pillow behind the knees to help ease the lower back closer to the floor. Do the same pillow propping when massaging the abdomen so the organs will be less constricted; and always move in a clockwise direction.

1. Make Contact.
2. Effleurage & Oiling.
3. Kneading.
4. Rib Circles.
5. Pectoral Effleurage.
6. Abdominal Cross-Stroke.
7. Abdominal Palm Circles.
8. Abdominal Traces.
9. Finger Pad Press Circles.
10. Cross Stroke
11. Final Effleurage.

V. *THE HANDS AND ARMS* often express how we feel. We extend our hand to shake "hello." We place an arm around someone's shoulder to give comfort or we reach out to embrace with affection. Like the face, they are expressive of our emotions and first to show age. If you want to massage someone who is really uncomfortable being touched, try the hands, for everyone is used to having them touched.

1. Pull & Shake.
2. Effleurage & Oiling.
3. Kneading.
4. Effleurage.
5. Pull & Shake.
6. Fingerpad Knead Hands.
7. Upper Arm Kneading.
8. Rolling.
9. Effleurage.
10. Arm Rotation.
11. Overhead Arm Stretch.

VI. *THE NECK, HEAD, AND FACE* is the area of the body where we feel most exposed to the world, and what we notice first in others. While joy shines out from bright eyes and a smile, a tight jaw and frown reveal anger and tension. Often this area is overlooked because it offers no large muscles to squeeze or manipulate. Take time to explore its curves, hollows, textures and bumps.

1. Cat's Paws.
2. Neck Stretch.
3. Effleurage and Oiling.
4. Small Friction Circles.
5. Side Effleurage.
6. Forward Stretch/Lift.
7. Scalp Circles.
8. Thumb Effleurage Forehead.
9. Eye Circles.
10. Eyelid Effleurage.
11. Nose Effleurage.
12. Sinus Press.
13. Lip Outline.
14. Cheek Knead.
15. Jaw Roll.
16. Ear Friction.
17. Ear Exploration.
18. Ear Hold.
19. Final Connecting Stroke.

use connecting strokes to integrate them and impart a sense of wholeness to the entire body. [Refer to video for massage instruction]

Massage for Everyone

You're never too young or too old to enjoy and benefit from massage. Whether you're trying to bond with your child, reduce stress, lose weight, or enhance your love life, massage has something for everyone.

Pregnant women appreciate being cared for during a time when all of their energy is directed toward nurturing the growth of a new being. Studies indicate that premature infants catch up in all aspects of their development when they're massaged in the first few months of life. Athletes who regularly get massaged improve their performance. And the elderly feel rejuvenated. Even pets respond favorably.

The massage techniques in "Massage for Health" are suitable for everyone as long as you take precautions for certain medical conditions (see CAUTION, p.13), and as long as you adjust the massage according to the needs of the individual you work on. For example, you would not give a runner a deep massage immediately before a race and of course, you would be very gentle with babies.

The following sections will help guide you in applying the massage instructions for the different kinds of people you might share massage with. By making the healing touch of massage an integral part of your life, you'll be practicing preventive health care right in your own home.

MASSAGE FOR THE WHOLE FAMILY

PREGNANCY

Pregnancy is a time to be pampered. The major changes that it generates in a woman's body and psyche call for special attention. Massage is a pleasurable way to express your love and support during those changes. And because a man doesn't physically experience the birth process, massage is an excellent opportunity for him to get more involved. Close friends and relatives may also want to massage the mother-to-be to demonstrate their caring during those nine months.

Midwives around the world have practiced prenatal massage for thousands of years. Today, in the developing countries, where they attend 60−80 percent of the births, it is still a valued tradition. If you were to visit a village in Guatemala or the Yucatan, you'd see that the custom of prenatal massage has hardly changed over the centuries. That's because women still appreciate the physical comfort and psychological reassurance that comes from the skillful touch of massage.

Prenatal massage has been practiced in Western medicine too. Not that long ago pregnancy alone was considered a contraindication for massage, but today doctors generally agree that massage is beneficial and safe provided certain precautions are taken. For example, if the woman has cardiac or circulatory problems, such as an embolism, it is unwise to massage her. Check with her obstetrician or midwife to be sure there are no conditions that massage could aggravate.

Doctors also advise not to massage vigorously on the abdomen or lower back/sacrum, because overly zealous handling can cause complications. And don't massage so deeply that the woman feels pain. Let her be your guide in how firm or soft your touch should be. If she is suddenly dizzy, nauseous, or uncomfortable in any other way, stop immediately. Have her sit up, drink a glass of water, or do whatever else will make her feel better. Continue only when she is okay again.

Massage feels good at any stage in a woman's life cycle, but perhaps even more so when she's preparing to bring a child into the world. Just being pregnant demands a lot of physical effort. All of a woman's systems are working twice as hard to sustain another being. The extra and unevenly distributed weight makes it more cumbersome to move. It distorts a woman's posture, causing discomfort and making it harder to rest for long. Massage can help reduce these difficulties.

Even if there are no specific aches, prenatal massage acts as an overall tonic. It also increases body awareness and gives the woman a chance to learn how to relax in preparation for labor. If she can't exercise, because of a heart condition or a history of miscarriages, massage is an alternative for stimulating circulation, stretching muscles, and keeping joints flexible.

You can easily adapt "Massage For Health" during pregnancy by keeping several things in mind. Most importantly, make sure the woman is comfortable. A pregnant woman tends to feel warmer than everyone else, so adjust the room temperature accordingly. Prop her with pillows and help her change positions as frequently as she finds necessary. When she's on her back, ease the strain in her lower back by placing a big pillow under her knees. In the later stages of pregnancy, lying supine for any length of time is not only uncomfortable, it can be dangerous. In this position, the baby lies directly on two major blood vessels, the dorsal aorta and inferior vena cava, and this could result in a fatal drop in blood pressure. To avoid this danger, have the *woman lie on her side instead.* Use extra pillows at her head, chest, belly, and between her legs, and pad her ankles with a folded towel. An alternative is to have her lean forward or back into a big pile of pillows on the floor.

You, too, need to be comfortable, so watch your own posture. Because you will be adjusting to new and different positions, take care in how you use your body to avoid any strain. Stop to shake out or stretch if you find yourself tensing up.

Massaging a pregnant woman also calls for improvising in the strokes you use and the sequence you follow. You won't be able to use all the movements in the instructions, nor do them in exactly the same order because the massage you give is dictated by the woman's comfort. If she can't lie down for long, don't try to force a whole body massage; do spot massages in a chair instead. If she can lie on her side, you can massage one whole side at a time. When doing the back, you might find it easier to start at the base of the spine and move up toward her shoulders. Then go to the hip and buttock, and finally the leg. In this postition, it's difficult to do the side-pulling effleurage with the forearm flat on the back. Instead, try a modified version from the front if the woman is comfortable lying on her back. Hook your hands under one side and pull them up, one after the other, but without coming across the whole front of the torso, as you would on the back. This feels especially good around the breasts, where pulling on a diagonal helps relieve pressure from their extra weight.

During the first six months of pregnancy, when a woman is still able to lie on her back, you can easily massage the abdomen. Although vigorous rubbing of the abdomen is unadvisable, slow and gentle clockwise circling of the belly with flat palms is soothing. Remember, you're now massaging two.

If the woman has moderate swelling in the arms and legs, you can help reduce it by promoting circulatory drainage with the V-effleurage. To relieve edema in the ankles, it's more effective to stroke the leg in a raised position, letting the foot rest on your shoulder, so gravity can assist in drainage. If she can't lie on her back, have her lean against some big pillows. Make deep, steady strokes up the thigh first, then up the lower leg, to create space in the tissue for the extra fluid to move into. If the feet are puffy, too, do them last. In a case of acute edema, don't try to massage it away. Instead, make sure she gets help from her midwife or obstetrician.

If you want to incorporate joint rotations, handle the woman's joints very carefully. By the end of the first three months, she experiences a surge of hormones that begin to loosen her ligaments. In the third trimester the hormone relaxin increases that loosening to prepare for the baby's passage through the pelvis, so don't yank or jerk.

If you're attentive to the expectant mother's needs and genuinely concerned for her well-being, she'll remember your massage as one of the highlights of her pregnancy. After childbirth is completed, you can continue to contribute significantly to this momentous event in a woman's life, for during postpartum recovery her body is still undergoing changes.

Postpartum massage is as much of a time-honored tradition as prenatal massage. In many agrarian cultures, peasant women rely on it to prepare them for working hard again. Among the Mayan Indians of Central America, massage also symbolically signals the end of a dangerous time for a woman and the lifting of restrictions placed on her during the critical period after birth. Among many women in Southeast Asia, especially Muslims in Malaysia and Indonesia, postpartum massage is considered essential to figure control.

For a postpartum massage, you can easily use the basic sequence in "Massage For Health." Pay special attention to the areas of the body that have been stressed the most, particularly the abdomen. Massage relieves the fatigue and tension incurred by the strenuous effort made during labor and delivery. It can also aid in strengthening muscles and preventing weakness due to inactivity, particularly for women who were confined during pregnancy and must convalesce afterward too. And whereas before birth hormones helped loosen a pregnant woman's body, now they're working to tighten things up again.

So, don't forget to give the same loving attention to a woman after she's given birth, especially if she suffers from postpartum depression. She'll greatly appreciate it as she works hard to get back in shape while devoting herself to the newborn child.

CHILDREN

We live in times that are rife with fear about the most negative form of touching—child abuse. Too many children are mistreated physically and sexually, and as a result, emotionally as well. The loving touch of massage is a positive way to assure that the next generation grows up with a foundation of trust and caring, which are vital in developing self-esteem.

Sharing massage with the youngest members of your family will add a whole new dimension to your relationship with them. Touch is a primary way to establish parent-infant bonding. In a sense, baby massage is a continuation of pregnancy massage outside the womb. Because touch is a baby's first major form of communication, children can quickly sense the message that's being conveyed when others touch them. All the more reason for setting a positive pattern right at the beginning.

Baby massage was revived in the West more than ten years ago, when Dr. Frederic Leboyer published *Loving Hands*, a photographic essay of a mother massaging her baby on the streets of Calcutta, India. Infant massage is a widespread practice in Asia, the Pacific Islands, and many other areas of the world, where it is generally part of the baby's bath routine. The massage is done by the mother, or other female relative, or even the midwife.

Massage helps infants grow healthy and strong and eat and sleep better. It also relieves colic, tummy aches, and other discomforts. Massaging premature babies enables them to catch up in their neurological, physical, mental and motor development. Children who are massaged often improve in behavior and schoolwork as they become more relaxed and less hyperactive. Historically, some cultures, like the Maoris and Hawaiians, have also used massage to correct deformed body parts and mold different features of the baby's body to attain their society's standards of beauty. They even massaged a child to prepare her for future activities, such as dancing.

In adapting "Massage for Health" for children, there are several considerations. Long before Dr. Leboyer, a pioneer in natural childbirth, suggested a soothing environment for babies, the ancient Greek physician Soranus advised that bathing and massaging a newborn calls for a small room which is moderately warm and without bright light.

Children have much less surface area to cover, so your movements will be much smaller. That also means it will take you less time to do a massage. This is a great advantage because most youngsters won't lie quiet for very long. A baby under four months old may tolerate only the briefest of massages and may want to suckle right away. When older babies and children start to move around, make a game out of the massage instead of trying to keep them still. Play with vibration and shaking movements. Create new names for any strokes you use. Children have vivid imaginations, so ask them what they see and feel inside as you're massaging them. If they're just learning vocabulary, you can use massage to teach them parts of the body.

Don't expect to do the same massage sequence or use the same pressure on your baby or toddler as you would on your partner. A lot of the massage will consist of light effleurage because it's the most soothing stroke, but you can also easily squeeze and wring the arms and legs. With bigger children, you can start on the back and add some of the strokes you would use on an adult body. You can also have them tell you which ones feel best.

In baby massage, it's better to start off on the front of the body. Let your baby lean against a big pillow or hold her in your lap. She'll feel safer if she can look at you, and her facial reactions will tell you how much pressure is comfortable.

On the baby's front, use your entire flat hands to start in the middle of the chest and spread outward in circles that reach the shoulders, come down the sides, and return to center. On the back, you can use one hand to support the baby at the buttocks or feet, while the other one—again, in a full, flat position—strokes up and down from the nape of the neck to the buttocks or vice versa. You can do the belly just as it was done during pregnancy, with gentle clockwise circing. For joint rotations, be sure your movements are moderate.

Massage is a great way to spend quality time with children, whether you're a hardworking parent with a busy schedule, a doting grandfather, or a favorite aunt. You'll feel a sense of satisfaction knowing you're giving them a headstart in developing personal relations based on mutual warmth and regard. As they develop strength and coordination, they can learn how to massage you as well. In fact, in most Asian countries it's customary for children to massage their elders. Now you can make it your custom too.

OLDER FOLKS

In traditional cultures, several generations live together, with each one performing an important role in the family. Grandparents, aunts and uncles help raise the children. That often includes the pleasant responsibility of massaging the youngsters from birth on. In turn, as the children grow, they massage those who cared for them.

In our highly mobile Western society, we tend to live far from our families, with generations separated from one another. But even when distance is not a barrier, we lead such hectic lives that we don't give enough time to the people who gave so much to us. Massage is an easy way to touch them with our love again.

The human need to be touched with caring doesn't diminish with age. Touch continues to contribute to our physical and emotional well-being long after its critical role in our survival as infants. In later years, massage can help assuage the isolation and loneliness we feel when we miss the people we've shared our lives with. Although reaching out to others is always a risk, the effort is well worth it, for giving and receiving massage revitalizes our connectedness to others, and can reaffirm our sense of identity and self-esteem. Even a simple hand or foot massage can make someone else, and you, feel better.

Massage provides physical stimulation to help ease certain conditions that often accompany growing older. Circulation slows down, the skin becomes thinner, the muscles have less tone, and the joints are less flexible. Rheumatism and arthritis lead to pain. Massage and joint rotation can increase circulation, mobilize the joints, and improve the condition of the skin. The relaxing effects of massage can also help lower blood pressure and relieve chronic tension headaches.

"Massage For Health" is ideal for older people as long as you are aware of their particular needs. If they have cardiovascular problems or joint inflammation due to arthritis, don't do massage. As with pregnant women and children, it's important to be sensitive to the unique condition of the older person you massage. Because you can't always follow the "Massage For Health" sequence to the letter, be flexible in adapting it for the person you work with. Learn to improvise.

If it's hard for older friends and relatives to lie down on or get up from the floor, have them relax in a chair. You can sit on the floor to do their legs, stand to work on their shoulders and head, have them lean forward on a pillow for a back massage, and rest their legs in your lap to do their feet. If they can lie down, be sure the surface is well padded, for bones become brittle as we age.

Unless you're massaging someone who is still physically strong and muscular, use light to medium pressure. Keeping extra blankets on hand will help avoid chilling. Or, you can have the person stay partially dressed, especially when seated in a chair.

Be patient and make the necessary adjustments. When you give of yourself through massage, you'll find the returns immeasurable. Remember that massage is a mutual experience at any age.

MASSAGE AND EXERCISE

Whether you're watching athletes right at a marathon, triathlon or cycling tour, or on TV, you can't help but notice the post-event massages they're treated to. Exercise and massage have been a winning combination ever since the ancient Greeks and Romans practiced them together. Athletes were massaged first to prepare them for action and later to relieve the fatigue and soreness produced by a vigorous workout, and also to help heal injuries. Today world-class athletes, including Olympic winners Edwin Moses and Joan Benoit, use massage for the same reasons. They want to increase their endurance and speed their recovery time so they can perform better.

But you and your partner don't have to be Olympic contenders to benefit from regular massage. Whether you jog your daily three miles or train for the Boston Marathon, play weekend tennis or aspire to Wimbledon, massage will make a noticeable difference. Added to a routine of stretching and warming up, it will promote greater flexibility. If you like to compete, but get nervous before a race, the relaxing effects of massage will help combat your anxiety. Massage will also lead to greater self-awareness. As you learn to recognize your body's signals, you'll be able to avoid overuse injuries, which result when you demand too much of your body too soon. If you do injure yourself, massage can help reduce the pain.

The instruction shared in "Massage For Health" is a bonus for anyone who is physically active. By taking into consideration who the person is, the kind of activity he engages in, and what the massage is intended for, you can adapt the techniques to best suit the exercise enthusiast you work. Remember, the condition of the athlete is what dictates the kind of massage you give.

If your partner has a light build, like Mary Decker Slaney, you won't work as hard on her as you would on her massive husband, discus-thrower Richard Slaney. You'll also focus on different sets of muscles, depending upon the individual's sport. If your partner is a swimmer, do more massage in the areas that receive the greatest workout: the trapezius muscles of the upper back and shoulders, the shoulder blades, the lower back, the arms, and the back of the thighs. For a cyclist, pay more attention to the legs. Keep in mind that although the quadriceps muscles (front of the thighs) are doing the most work, the hamstrings (back of the thighs) are taking a beating because they're constantly shortening. You can help stretch and loosen them with a combination of vibration, friction and kneading. Because of their hunched-forward position, cyclists are also susceptible to wrist strains and forearm cramping, as well as lower back and shoulder aches, so don't forget these fatigue areas either.

If you want to give someone a boost right before exercise, make sure your massage is stimulating. A slow, soothing massage could relax your partner so much he won't feel energetic enough to go out and do his best. Briskly apply effleurage and percussion, especially to the parts of the body that will be used most. This will help bring oxygen to the muscles immediately. Gentle joint rotations will also help with flexibility. A tennis player will need it the most in the shoulders, elbows and wrists. A basketball player will also appreciate it in the hips, knees and ankles.

If you work with an athlete one or two days before an event, you can do a deeper, more conditioning massage using kneading and friction strokes. Again, pay extra attention to the muscle groups and joints that will be stressed. To prepare a runner for a meet, use friction to spread the muscle fibers in the calves and thighs to allow for greater oxygen capacity, and throughly work the foot, for it will take a lot of punishment, especially on hard surfaces. A foot massage alone can do wonders to help someone feel better overall, for the feet, which we use in every sport, have nerve endings that connect to all parts of the body.

Right after strenuous exercise an athlete's pain tolerance is lower, so don't massage vigorously. Muscles might cramp in response to deep strokes. Work more slowly and gradually to have a relaxing effect. If your partner can't handle any pressure, it's best to first loosen up the muscles with some shaking and vibration. for example, after a long-distance race, most runners would rather have you shake out their calves, which you can do by holding the foot, with the knee bent. Then lower the leg and use effleurage and kneading to stimulate removal of metabolic by-products such as lactic acid, which cause soreness and fatigue. When massaging the limbs, direct the pressure toward the heart. Increased circulation will bring fresh nutrients like oxygen to the muscles, replenishing their energy supply. And be sure your partner is warm enough; chilled muscles can't relax.

If you want to help your partner when she's already been hurt, it's essential that you know your limits. *Don't massage a freshly injured area*, especially a fracture or dislocation, because pressure and movement can aggravate the damage. It's safer to start off with RICE (rest, ice, compression, and elevation) and consult a doctor. With medical advice, you may be able to massage within 24 to 48 hours to help speed recovery from sprains, strains, tendon or ligament tears.

One of the best ways you can assist your partner's healing is by reducing swelling in the limbs. The extra fluid leads to pressure and stiffness, making movement painful. Massage stimulates circulation to carry it away and bring in vital nutrients that promote healing. In order to make room for the fluid to leave the injured area—let's say a hand or wrist that's been sprained in a baseball or basketball game—you need to effleurage first the upper arm, which is closest to the heart, then the lower arm. Keeping the arm raised while you do this will give gravity a chance to assist drainage.

Once swelling goes down, generally soreness leaves and normal motion is restored, allowing activity once again. This is important in the long run because moving sooner reduces the likelihood that restrictive scar tissue will form in the injured muscle during the healing period. When transverse adhesions, rather than strong longitudinal scars, form, the muscle fibers join together or to bone. This kind of fibrous tissue is weaker, chronically painful, and susceptible to re-injury. Cross-fiber friction can help inhibit formation of adhesions, or break them down once formed. To be most effective, consult a medical professional so that you know exactly where to apply the friction and in which direction you should be doing the stroke to help separate the fibers.

While massage is advantageous in improving overall athletic performance and preventing injuries, it may help the most zealous of exercise buffs in a way they'd least consider. For those people who are relentlessly competitive, it's essential to take time out to be passive, to take a real body/mind break and completely relax. Giving up control of your muscles for just a little while will give you the opportunity to experience your next run, ride, or game with more pleasure and without pain.

SHARI BELAFONTE

In a professional career that spans a few short years, beautiful and vivacious Shari Belafonte has achieved great success in a career that includes modeling, acting and singing. Daughter of acclaimed entertainer Harry Belafonte, Shari has graced over 200 magazine covers, is currently a series co-star on ABC-TV's "Hotel," and has released a top selling album in Europe. A natural athlete and health enthusiast, Shari enjoys jogging, cycling, aerobics and dance. Massage was introduced to Shari while working in Japan in 1982, and it has since become an integral part of her active lifestyle.

MIRKA KNASTER, M.A.

Mirka Knaster has been a massage therapist/instructor and wholistic health educator since 1978. She has given numerous classes, workshops and lecture/demonstrations for schools, health fairs, resorts, runners' clubs, and psychotherapy groups. Based on her private practice, teaching experiences and many years of cross-cultural research, Mirka writes regularly about massage and the importance of touch. A contributing editor for EAST WEST JOURNAL and former columnist for MASSAGE MAGAZINE, Mirka has had articles in numerous publications, including THE WASHINGTON POST, BETTER HEALTH AND LIVING, and WOMEN'S HEALTH CARE: A GUIDE TO ALTERNATIVES.

JAMES HEARTLAND

James Heartland is currently in private practice teaching massage at the Tao of Healing Arts in Santa Monica, California. James has been trained and certified in Jin Shin Do Acupressure, Reichian Therapy and Sports Massage, and was part of the sports massage team for the Los Angeles Triathlon and the 1984 Olympic Games.

ACKNOWLEDGEMENTS

Healing Arts Home Video extends warm appreciation to the following individuals:

Lois Adams, Louis Almeida, Sally Altabet, Catherine Bension, Sam Bercholtz, Jeff Blair, Lois Blair, Craig Blankenhorn, Bob Crawford, Dom Deluise, Joel Dweck, Inger Jensen, Maria Joseph, Do Ahn Kaneko, John Kemp, Krishna Kaur Khalsa, Marjorie Kwawer, Judy Lamm, Gabe Lesky, Bob Maile, Kathleen Mulchay, Anne Reeves, Mamoru Shimokochi, Terry Unger, Twinka Thiebaud.

For additional information or comments write:
"Massage For Health," Healing Arts Publishing, Inc.,
321 Hampton Drive, Ste. 203, Venice, CA 90291

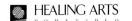

HEALING ARTS
HOME VIDEO